COMPLETE EASY 30 MINUTES HEART HEALTHY COOKBOOK

GEORGE ANDERSON

CHAPTER ONE

INTRODUCTION

Heart

The heart is a muscular organ in most animals. This organ pumps blood through the blood vessels of the circulatory system. The pumped blood carries oxygen and nutrients to the body, while carrying metabolic waste such as carbon dioxide to the lungs. In humans, the heart is approximately the size of a closed fist and is located between the lungs, in the middle compartment of the chest.

In humans, other mammals, and birds, the heart is divided into four chambers: upper left and right atria and lower left and right ventricles. Commonly the right atrium and ventricle are referred together as the right heart and their left counterparts as the left heart. Fish, in contrast, have two chambers, an atrium and a ventricle, while most reptiles have three chambers. In a healthy heart blood flows one way through the heart due to heart valves, which prevent backflow. The heart is enclosed in a protective sac, the pericardium, which also contains a small amount of fluid. The wall of the heart is made up of three layers: epicardium, myocardium, and endocardium.

The heart pumps blood with a rhythm determined by a group of pacemaker cells in the sinoatrial node. These generate a current that causes the heart to contract, traveling through the atrioventricular node and along the conduction system of the heart. In humans, deoxygenated blood enters the heart through the right atrium from the superior and inferior venae cavae and passes it to the right ventricle. From here it is pumped into pulmonary circulation to the lungs, where it receives oxygen and gives off carbon dioxide. Oxygenated blood then returns to the left atrium, passes through the left ventricle and is pumped out through the aorta into systemic circulation, traveling through arteries, arterioles, and capillaries where nutrients and other substances are exchanged between blood vessels and cells, losing oxygen and gaining carbon dioxide before being returned to the heart through venules and veins. The heart beats at a resting rate close to 72 beats per minute. Exercise temporarily increases the rate, but lowers resting heart rate in the long term, and is good for heart health.

Cardiovascular diseases (CVD) are the most common cause of death globally as of 2008, accounting for 30% of deaths. Of these more than three-quarters are a result of coronary artery disease and stroke. Risk factors include: smoking, being overweight, little exercise, high cholesterol, high blood pressure, and poorly controlled diabetes, among others. Cardiovascular diseases frequently do not have symptoms or may cause chest pain or shortness of breath. Diagnosis of heart disease is often done by the taking of a medical history, listening to the heart-sounds with a stethoscope, ECG, echocardiogram, and ultrasound. Specialists who focus on diseases of the heart are called cardiologists, although many specialties of medicine may be involved in treatment.

INCREDIBLY HEART-HEALTHY FOODS

Heart disease accounts for nearly one-third of all deaths worldwide.

Diet plays a major role in heart health and can impact your risk of heart disease.

In fact, certain foods can influence blood pressure, triglycerides, cholesterol levels and inflammation, all of which are risk factors for heart disease.

Here are 15 foods that you should be eating to maximize your heart health.

1. Leafy green vegetables

Leafy green vegetables like spinach, kale, and collard greens are well known for their wealth of vitamins, minerals, and antioxidants.

In particular, they're a great source of vitamin K, which helps protect your arteries and promote proper blood clotting.

They're also high in dietary nitrates, which have been shown to reduce blood pressure, decrease arterial stiffness, and improve the function of cells lining the blood vessels.

Some studies have also found a link between increasing your intake of leafy green vegetables and a lower risk of heart disease.

One analysis of eight studies found that increasing leafy green vegetable intake was associated with up to a 16% lower incidence of heart disease.

Another study in 29,689 women showed that a high intake of leafy green vegetables was linked to a significantly lower risk of coronary heart disease.

2. Whole grains

Whole grains include all three nutrient-rich parts of the grain:

- germ

- endosperm

- bran

Common types of whole grains include:

- whole wheat

- brown rice

- oats

- rye

- barley

- buckwheat

- quinoa

Refined carbohydrates increase the risk of coronary heart disease. Conversely, whole grains are protective. An extra 1 or 2 servings per day of these foods increases or decreases risk by approximately 10% to 20%.

Multiple studies have found that including more whole grains in your diet can benefit your heart health.

One analysis of 45 studies concluded that eating three more servings of whole grains daily was associated with a 22% lower risk of heart disease.

Adopting a diet rich in plant-based foods, whole grains, low fat dairy products, and sodium intake within normal limits can be effective in the prevention and management of hypertension.

When purchasing whole grains, make sure to read the ingredients label carefully. Phrases like "whole grain" or "whole wheat" indicate a whole grain product, while words like "wheat flour" or "multigrain" may not.

3. Berries

Strawberries, blueberries, blackberries, and raspberries are jam-packed with important nutrients that play a central role in heart health.

Berries are also rich in antioxidants like anthocyanins, which protect against the oxidative stress and inflammation that contribute to the development of heart disease.

Studies show that eating lots of berries can reduce several risk factors for heart disease.

For example, one study in 33 adults with obesity showed that consuming strawberries at two and a half servings for 4 weeks significantly improved insulin resistance and LDL (bad) cholesterol.

Another study found that eating blueberries daily improved the function of cells that line the blood vessels, which help control blood pressure and blood clotting.

Additionally, an analysis of 22 studies showed that eating berries was associated with reductions in LDL (bad) cholesterol, systolic blood pressure, body mass index, and certain markers of inflammation.

Berries can be a satisfying snack or delicious low calorie dessert. Try adding a few different types to your diet to take advantage of their unique health benefits.

4. Avocados

Avocados are an excellent source of heart-healthy monounsaturated fats, which have been linked to reduced levels of cholesterol and a lower risk of heart disease.

One study looked at the effects of three cholesterol-lowering diets in 45 people with overweight and obesity, with one of the test groups consuming one avocado per day.

The avocado group experienced reductions in LDL (bad) cholesterol, including lower levels of small, dense LDL (bad) cholesterol, which is believed to significantly raise the risk of heart disease.

The lipid-lowering and cardioprotective effects of avocado have been demonstrated in several studies.

Avocados are also rich in potassium, a nutrient that's essential to heart health. In fact, just one avocado supplies 975 milligrams of potassium, or about 28% of the amount that you need in a day.

Getting at least 4.7 grams of potassium per day can decrease blood pressure by an average of 8.0/4.1 mmHg, which is associated with a 15% lower risk of stroke.

5. Fatty fish and fish oil

Fatty fish like salmon, mackerel, sardines, and tuna are loaded with omega-3 fatty acids, which have been studied extensively for their heart-health benefits.

Omega-3 fatty acids from fatty fish may have a protective role in the risk of developing heart disease and slightly reduce the risk of CVD events and arrhythmias.

Another study showed that eating fish over the long term was linked to lower levels of total cholesterol, blood triglycerides, fasting blood sugar, and systolic blood pressure.

Fish consumption is associated with a lower risk of cardiovascular disease, depression, and mortality.

If you don't eat much seafood, fish oil is another option for getting your daily dose of omega-3 fatty acids.

Fish oil supplements have been shown to reduce blood triglycerides, improve arterial function, and decrease blood pressure.

Other omega-3 supplements like krill oil or algal oil are popular alternatives.

6. Walnuts

Walnuts are a great source of fiber and micronutrients like magnesium, copper, and manganese.

Research shows that incorporating a few servings of walnuts in your diet can help protect against heart disease.

Evidence for cardiovascular disease prevention is strong for some varieties of tree nuts, particularly walnuts.

A 2009 study in 365 participants showed that diets supplemented with walnuts led to greater decreases in LDL (bad) and total cholesterol.

Interestingly, some studies have also found that regularly eating nuts such as walnuts is associated with a lower risk of heart disease.

7. Beans

Beans contain resistant starch, which resists digestion and is fermented by the beneficial bacteria in your gut. Resistant starch has the potential to exert a healthy impact on the gut and certain members of its resident microbiota.

Multiple studies have also found that eating beans can reduce certain risk factors for heart disease.

In an older study of 16 people, eating pinto beans reduced levels of blood triglycerides and LDL (bad) cholesterol.

One review of 26 studies also found that a diet high in beans and legumes significantly decreased levels of LDL (bad) cholesterol.

What's more, eating beans has been linked to reduced blood pressure and inflammation, both of which are risk factors for heart disease.

8. Dark chocolate

Dark chocolate is rich in antioxidants like flavonoids, which can help boost heart health.

Interestingly, several studies have associated eating chocolate with a lower risk of heart disease.

Consuming chocolate in moderation (less than 6 servings a week) may decrease your risk of coronary heart disease, stroke, and diabetes.

Keep in mind that these studies show an association but don't necessarily account for other factors that may be involved.

Additionally, chocolate can be high in sugar and calories, which can negate many of its health-promoting properties.

Be sure to pick a high quality dark chocolate with a cocoa content of at least 70% and moderate your intake to make the most of its heart-healthy benefits.

9. Tomatoes

Tomatoes are loaded with lycopene, a natural plant pigment with powerful antioxidant properties.

Antioxidants help neutralize harmful free radicals, preventing oxidative damage and inflammation, both of which can contribute to heart disease.

Low blood levels of lycopene are linked to an increased risk of heart attack and stroke.

Increasing the intake of tomato products and lycopene supplementation have positive effects on blood lipids, blood pressure, and endothelial function.

Another study in 50 women with overweight found that eating two raw tomatoes four times per week increased levels of HDL (good) cholesterol.

Higher levels of HDL (good) cholesterol can help remove excess cholesterol and plaque from the arteries to keep your heart healthy and protect against heart disease and stroke.

10. Almonds

Almonds are incredibly nutrient-dense, boasting a long list of vitamins and minerals that are crucial to heart health.

They're also a good source of heart-healthy monounsaturated fats and fiber, two important nutrients that can help protect against heart disease.

Research suggests that eating almonds can have a powerful effect on your cholesterol levels, too.

One study involving 48 people with high cholesterol showed that eating 1.5 ounces (43 grams) of almonds daily for 6 weeks reduced belly fat and levels of LDL (bad) cholesterol, two risk factors for heart disease.

Research also shows that eating almonds is associated with higher levels of HDL (good) cholesterol, which can help reduce plaque buildup and keep your arteries clear.

Remember that while almonds are very high in nutrients, they're also high in calories. Measure your portions and moderate your intake if you're trying to lose weight.

11. Seeds

Chia seeds, flaxseeds, and hemp seeds are all great sources of heart-healthy nutrients, including fiber and omega-3 fatty acids.

Numerous studies have found that adding these types of seeds to your diet can improve many heart disease risk factors, including inflammation, blood pressure, cholesterol, and triglycerides.

For example, hemp seeds are high in arginine, an amino acid that has been associated with reduced blood levels of certain inflammatory markers.

Furthermore, flaxseed may help keep blood pressure and cholesterol levels well managed.

Supplementing your diet with milled flaxseed has many health-promoting benefits for the body. There is evidence that dietary flaxseed lowers your risk of cardiovascular disease and cancer, and may help other conditions like gastrointestinal health and diabetes.

Chia seeds are another great food source for heart health. Although more research is needed about the effects of chia seeds on heart health in humans, one study in rats found that eating chia seeds lowered blood triglyceride levels and boosted levels of beneficial HDL (good) cholesterol.

12. Garlic

For centuries, garlic has been used as a natural remedy to treat a variety of ailments.

In recent years, research has confirmed its potent medicinal properties and found that garlic can even help improve heart health.

This is thanks to the presence of a compound called allicin, which is believed to have a multitude of therapeutic effects.

In one study, taking garlic extract in doses of 600–1,500 mg daily for 24 weeks was as effective as a common prescription drug at reducing blood pressure.

One review compiled the results of 39 studies and found that garlic can reduce total cholesterol by an average of 17 mg/dL and LDL (bad) cholesterol by 9 mg/dL in those with high cholesterol.

Other studies have found that garlic extract can inhibit platelet buildup, which may reduce the risk of blood clots and stroke.

Be sure to consume garlic raw, or crush it and let it sit for a few minutes before cooking. This allows for the formation of allicin, maximizing its potential health benefits.

13. Olive oil

A staple in the Mediterranean diet, the heart-healthy benefits of olive oil are well documented.

Olive oil is packed with antioxidants, which can relieve inflammation and decrease the risk of chronic disease.

It's also rich in monounsaturated fatty acids, which many studies have associated with improvements in heart health.

In fact, one study involving 7,216 adults at high risk for heart disease showed that those who consumed the most olive oil had a 35% lower risk of developing heart disease.

Furthermore, a higher intake of olive oil was associated with a 48% lower risk of dying from heart disease.

Olive oil is high in oleic acid and antioxidants, and has been found to be helpful at preventing and treating hypertension.

Take advantage of the many benefits of olive oil by drizzling it over cooked dishes or adding it to vinaigrettes and sauces.

14. Edamame

Edamame is an immature soybean frequently found in Asian cuisine.

Like other soy products, edamame is rich in soy isoflavones, a type of flavonoid that may help lower cholesterol levels and improve heart health.

Including soy protein in your diet may lead to a reduced risk of cardiovascular disease.

If combined with other changes to diet and lifestyle, even slightly reducing your cholesterol levels can have a big impact on your risk of heart disease.

One study showed that including 30 grams of soy protein per day in a lipid-lowering diet improved participants' blood lipids, reducing the risk for cardiovascular disease.

In addition to its isoflavone content, edamame is a good source of other heart-healthy nutrients, including dietary fiber and antioxidants.

15. Green tea

Green tea has been associated with a number of health benefits, from increased fat burning to improved insulin sensitivity.

It's also brimming with polyphenols and catechins, which can act as antioxidants to prevent cell damage, reduce inflammation, and protect the health of your heart.

One study showed that green tea extract effectively increased leptin and reduced LDL (bad) cholesterol in women with overweight and obesity after 6 weeks of treatment even though there were no significant changes in other biochemical markers related to weight.

A review of studies found that taking green tea extract for 3 months reduced blood pressure, triglycerides, LDL (bad) and total cholesterol, compared to a placebo.

Taking a green tea supplement or drinking matcha, a beverage that is similar to green tea but made with the whole tea leaf, may also benefit heart health.

CHAPTER TWO

A 3-DAY HEART-HEALTHY MENU

If you're concerned about your heart health and want to follow a healthier diet in order to reduce your risk of cardiovascular disease, there are simple ways to make your diet more heart-healthy.

For example, adding more fiber into your diet by increasing your intake of fiber-rich foods like fruits, vegetables, and beans is an easy and delicious way to improve heart health.

Here's a 3-day heart-healthy meal plan to help get you started.

Day 1

- Breakfast: an egg omelet made with sautéed peppers, kale, and onions served with sliced avocado and berries

- Lunch: lentil soup served with a green salad with pumpkin seeds, feta cheese, cherry tomatoes, and olive oil and balsamic vinaigrette

- Dinner: salmon with pesto served with broccoli and roasted sweet potatoes

- Snacks: trail mix made with almonds, cashews, sunflower seeds, and dried cherries

Day 2

- Breakfast: overnight oats made with almond butter, chia seeds, cashew milk, golden raisins, and mixed berries

- Lunch: Mediterranean quinoa salad, with arugula, chickpeas, sun-dried tomatoes, roasted red peppers, olives, and feta cheese with an olive oil and balsamic vinaigrette

- Dinner: baked chicken breast with butternut squash and asparagus

- Snacks: unsweetened Greek yogurt with diced apples, sliced almonds, and cinnamon

Day 3

- Breakfast: shakshuka a Mediterranean-style breakfast made with eggs and tomatoes served with a slice of sprouted grain bread topped with mashed avocado and chili flakes

- Lunch: grilled shrimp and pineapple kabobs over a large green salad with an olive oil and herb vinaigrette

- Dinner: black bean burgers served with cucumber and red onion salad and roasted herbed potato wedges

- Snacks: garlic hummus with fresh vegetable sticks

Following a diet rich in nutrient-dense foods like the ones above while limiting foods and beverages associated with negative heart health outcomes can help keep your cardiovascular system healthy and reduce your risk of heart disease.

OTHER DIET AND LIFESTYLE TIPS THAT MAY SUPPORT HEART HEALTH

Whether you want to support treatment for an existing heart disease or reduce your risk of developing heart disease, there are many simple ways to protect your cardiovascular system through diet and lifestyle modification.

Here are some evidence-based diet and lifestyle tips for heart health.

Quit smoking

Smoking significantly increases your risk of developing heart disease and can worsen heart disease symptoms. If you currently smoke, consider quitting.

If you need help and resources to do so, visit smokefree.gov.

Eat more fiber-rich plant foods

Diets high in fiber have been linked to improved heart health and decreased heart disease risk. Try eating more high-fiber foods like fruits, vegetables, nuts, seeds, and whole grains.

Sit less and move more

Leading a sedentary lifestyle could increase your risk of developing heart disease. Make an effort to sit less and move more, if you can, by going for regular walks or engaging in other exercise you enjoy.

Switch to healthier fats

Fats are satisfying and make meals taste delicious. Focus on eating more sources of healthy fat like olive oil, avocados, nuts, seeds, nut butter, and fatty fish.

Consider supplements

Studies show that certain dietary supplements specifically fish oil and magnesium may help lower heart disease risk, especially for those with heart disease risk factors like type 2 diabetes and high blood pressure.

Limit certain foods and beverages

Some foods and drinks like fast food, sugary beverages (such as soda), processed meats, and refined grains appear to negatively affect heart health.

Do your best to consume these only in small amounts, especially if you're at risk of developing heart disease.

Manage stress

Chronic stress negatively affects the body in many ways and may even increase the risk of heart disease. Learning ways to manage or relieve stress whenever possible is a smart way to care for your heart.

In addition to the tips listed above, there are many other ways to protect your heart health, including getting enough sleep and limiting your alcohol intake.

HEART HEALTHY RECIPES

Here are some recipes I explained here that are very good for your heart, each recipes are explained by listing the ingredients and the instructions of prepartions

Salmon with Chopped Tomatillo Salad

Ingredients

- 1 ¼ pounds salmon fillet, cut into 4 portions

- 2 tablespoons extra-virgin olive oil, divided

- ¾ teaspoon kosher salt, divided

- ½ teaspoon ground pepper, divided

- ½ teaspoon ground cumin

- 8 ounces tomatillos, husked, rinsed and chopped (see Tip)

- 1 medium tomato, chopped

- ½ cup chopped fresh cilantro

- ½ cup chopped red onion

- 1 medium jalapeño pepper, chopped

- 2 tablespoons lime juice

Directions

- Step 1

Position rack in upper third of oven; preheat broiler to high.

- Step 2

Place salmon on a rimmed baking sheet. Drizzle with 1 tablespoon oil and sprinkle with 1/2 teaspoon salt, 1/4 teaspoon pepper and cumin. Broil the salmon until it is opaque and flakes easily with a fork, 6 to 9 minutes.

- Step 3

Meanwhile, combine tomatillos, tomato, cilantro, onion, jalapeño and lime juice with the remaining 1 tablespoon oil and 1/4 teaspoon each salt and pepper in a medium bowl. Serve the salmon with the salad.

Black Beans & Corn with Poached Eggs

Ingredients

- 2 tablespoons olive oil

- 1 medium onion, diced

- 1 red bell pepper, diced

- ½ cup corn kernels (frozen or fresh)

- 4 cloves garlic, chopped

- ½ jalapeño pepper, seeded and minced

- 1 teaspoon ground cumin

- 1 teaspoon dried oregano

- 1 (15 ounce) can low-sodium black beans, rinsed

- 1 (4 ounce) can chopped green chiles

- 1 teaspoon red-wine vinegar

- ½ teaspoon salt

- 4 large eggs

- ¼ cup chopped fresh cilantro

- 2 tablespoons crumbled queso fresco or feta cheese

- 2 tablespoons minced red onion

Directions

- Step 1

Heat oil in a 10-inch skillet over medium heat. Add onion, bell pepper, corn, garlic, jalapeño, cumin, and oregano. Cook, stirring often, until the onions are translucent and the spices are fragrant, about 5 minutes. Stir in beans, chiles, vinegar, and salt; cook, stirring, for 2 minutes.

- Step 2

Use a spoon to make 4 indentations in the bean mixture. Crack an egg into each indentation. Cover and cook until the whites are set but yolks are still runny, 4 to 6 minutes (or until desired doneness).

- Step 3

Sprinkle with cilantro, queso fresco (or feta), and red onion and serve.

Herby Fish with Wilted Greens & Mushrooms

Ingredients

- 3 tablespoons olive oil, divided

- ½ large sweet onion, sliced

- 3 cups sliced cremini mushrooms

- 2 cloves garlic, sliced

- 4 cups chopped kale

- 1 medium tomato, diced

- 2 teaspoons Mediterranean Herb Mix (see Associated Recipes), divided

- 1 tablespoon lemon juice

- ½ teaspoon salt, divided

- ½ teaspoon ground pepper, divided

- 4 (4 ounce) cod, sole, or tilapia fillets

- Chopped fresh parsley, for garnish

Directions

- Step 1

Heat 1 Tbsp. oil in a large saucepan over medium heat. Add onion; cook, stirring occasionally, until translucent, 3 to 4 minutes. Add mushrooms and garlic; cook, stirring occasionally, until the mushrooms release their liquid and begin to brown, 4 to 6 minutes. Add kale, tomato, and 1 tsp. herb mix. Cook, stirring occasionally, until the kale is wilted and the mushrooms are tender, 5 to 7 minutes. Stir in lemon juice and 1/4 tsp. each salt and pepper. Remove from heat, cover, and keep warm.

- Step 2

Sprinkle fish with the remaining 1 tsp. herb mix and 1/4 tsp. each salt and pepper. Heat the remaining 2 Tbsp. oil in a large nonstick skillet over medium-high heat. Add the fish and cook until the flesh is opaque, 2 to 4 minutes per side, depending on thickness. Transfer the fish to 4 plates or a serving platter. Top and surround the fish with the vegetables; sprinkle with parsley, if desired.

Vegan Black Bean Burgers

Ingredients

- 1 (15.5 ounce) can no-salt-added black beans, rinsed

- 1 cup cooked quinoa

- ½ cup whole-wheat panko breadcrumbs

- ½ cup chopped scallions

- 1 tablespoon no-salt-added tomato paste

- 1 ½ teaspoons ground cumin

- ½ teaspoon chipotle chile powder

- ½ teaspoon garlic powder

- ½ cup vegan mayonnaise, divided

- ½ teaspoon salt, divided

- 1 medium avocado

- 2 tablespoons lime juice

- 2 tablespoons chopped fresh cilantro

- 2 tablespoons water

- 2 tablespoons extra-virgin olive oil

- 6 small whole-wheat hamburger buns, toasted

- 6 thin slices tomato

Directions

- Step 1

Place beans, quinoa, panko, scallions, tomato paste, cumin, chile powder, garlic powder, 1/4 cup mayonnaise and 1/4 teaspoon salt in a large bowl; mash the mixture together with your hands. Shape into six 3/4-inch-thick patties. Arrange the patties on a plate; refrigerate for 10 minutes.

- Step 2

Combine avocado, lime juice, cilantro, water and the remaining 1/4 cup mayonnaise and 1/4 teaspoon salt in a food processor; process until smooth, about 30 seconds.

- Step 3

Heat oil in a large cast-iron skillet over medium-high heat. Add the patties; cook until golden brown, 3 to 4 minutes per side.

- Step 4

Divide the avocado mixture evenly among top and bottom bun halves. Arrange the bean patties and tomato slices evenly on the bottom bun halves; replace the top bun halves.

Cheeseburger Stuffed Baked Potatoes

Ingredients

- 4 medium russet potatoes (about 8 ounces each)

- ½ cup low-fat mayonnaise

- 8 ounces cooked ground beef, warmed

- ½ cup shredded iceberg lettuce

- ½ cup diced tomato

- ¼ cup sliced red onion

- 4 teaspoons shredded Colby Jack cheese

Directions

- Step 1

Pierce potatoes all over with a fork. Microwave on Medium, turning once or twice, until soft, about 20 minutes. (Alternatively, bake potatoes at 425 degrees F until tender, 45 minutes to 1 hour.) Transfer to a clean cutting board and let cool slightly.

- Step 2

Holding them with a kitchen towel to protect your hands, make a lengthwise cut to open the potato, but don't cut all the way through. Pinch the ends to expose the flesh.

- Step 3

Top each potato with some mayonnaise, beef, lettuce, tomato, red onion and cheese. Serve warm.

Grilled Salmon with Cilantro-Ginger Sauce

Ingredients

Cilantro-Ginger Sauce

- 1 tablespoon toasted sesame oil

- 1 tablespoon fresh lime juice

- 1 tablespoon chopped fresh cilantro

- 1 teaspoon fish sauce

- 1 teaspoon minced seeded Thai red chile (about 1 large) or jalapeño pepper

- 1 teaspoon grated fresh ginger

- 1 teaspoon honey

- 1 medium clove garlic, mashed into paste

Salmon

- 1 pound skin-on salmon fillet (about 2 inches thick), preferably wild-caught, cut into 4 portions

- 1 tablespoon toasted sesame oil

- ½ teaspoon ground pepper

- ¼ teaspoon salt

Directions

- Step 1

To prepare sauce: Whisk oil, lime juice, cilantro, fish sauce, chile (or jalapeño), ginger, honey, and garlic in a small bowl. Reserve 1 Tbsp. of the sauce in a separate small bowl to use for basting.

- Step 2

To prepare salmon: Preheat grill to medium-high (see Tip). Pat salmon dry with paper towels. Rub oil all over the salmon. Sprinkle both sides with pepper and salt. Place the salmon on the grill, skin-side up. Grill until the salmon lifts from the grates without sticking, about 6 minutes. Flip the salmon and brush with the reserved 1 Tbsp. sauce. Cook until the salmon lifts from the grates without sticking and flakes with a fork, 1 to 2 minutes more. Serve with the remaining sauce.

Shrimp & Pepper Kebabs with Grilled Red Onion Slaw

Ingredients

- ½ cup chopped fresh parsley

- ⅓ cup chopped scallions

- ⅓ cup crumbled feta cheese

- 3 tablespoons red-wine vinegar

- ⅓ cup canola oil plus 1 tablespoon, divided

- 1 pound raw shrimp (21-25 count), peeled and deveined

- 24 mini bell peppers (15 ounces)

- 1 small red onion, cut into quarters

- 1 (10 ounce) package coleslaw mix (with carrots and red cabbage)

- 1 ½ cups pita chips, crushed

Directions

- Step 1

Preheat grill to medium-high.

- Step 2

Place parsley, scallions, feta, vinegar and 1/3 cup oil in a mini food processor; blend until mostly smooth. Set aside.

- Step 3

Thread 3 shrimp and 3 mini peppers on each of 8 bamboo skewers. Brush the kebabs and onion with the remaining 1 tablespoon oil. Grill the kebabs until the shrimp turn pink and are opaque in the center and the peppers are lightly charred, about 3 minutes per side. Grill the onion wedges until slightly softened and charred, 2 to 3 minutes per side. Remove from the grill.

- Step 4

Reserve 1/4 cup of the dressing. Combine slaw mix, pita chips and the remaining dressing in a large bowl. When the onion is cool enough to handle, thinly slice and toss with the slaw mixture.

- Step 5

Serve the slaw and kebabs with the reserved dressing.

Mushroom & Tofu Stir-Fry

Ingredients

- 4 tablespoons peanut oil or canola oil, divided

- 1 pound mixed mushrooms, sliced

- 1 medium red bell pepper, diced

- 1 bunch scallions, trimmed and cut into 2-inch pieces

- 1 tablespoon grated fresh ginger

- 1 large clove garlic, grated

- 1 (8 ounce) container baked tofu or smoked tofu, diced

- 3 tablespoons oyster sauce or vegetarian oyster sauce (see Tip)

Directions

- Step 1

Heat 2 tablespoons oil in a large flat-bottom wok or cast-iron skillet over high heat. Add mushrooms and bell pepper; cook, stirring occasionally, until soft, about 4 minutes. Stir in scallions, ginger and garlic; cook for 30 seconds more. Transfer the vegetables to a bowl.

- Step 2

Add the remaining 2 tablespoons oil and tofu to the pan. Cook, turning once, until browned, 3 to 4 minutes. Stir in the vegetables and oyster sauce. Cook, stirring, until hot, about 1 minute.

Beef Stir-Fry with Baby Bok Choy & Ginger

Ingredients

- 12 ounces beef flank steak, trimmed

- 1 tablespoon minced fresh ginger

- 1 ½ teaspoons reduced-sodium soy sauce

- 1 teaspoon dry sherry plus 1 Tbsp., divided

- 1 teaspoon cornstarch

- 1 teaspoon toasted sesame oil

- 2 tablespoons oyster-flavored sauce, preferably Lee Kum Kee Premium

- 1 tablespoon vegetable oil

- 1 pound baby bok choy, trimmed and cut into 2-inch pieces (about 8 cups)

- 3 tablespoons unsalted chicken broth

Directions

- Step 1

Cut beef with the grain into 2-inch-wide strips. Cut each strip across the grain into 1/4-inch-thick slices. Combine the beef, ginger, soy sauce, 1 tsp. sherry, and cornstarch in a medium bowl; stir until the cornstarch is no longer visible. Add sesame oil and stir until the beef is lightly coated.

- Step 2

Combine oyster-flavored sauce and the remaining 1 Tbsp. sherry in a small bowl. Set aside.

- Step 3

Heat a 14-inch flat-bottomed carbon-steel wok (or a 12-inch stainless-steel skillet) over high heat until a drop of water vaporizes within 1 to 2 seconds of contact. Swirl in vegetable oil. Add the beef in an even layer; cook, undisturbed, until it begins to brown, about 1 minute. Using a metal spatula, stir-fry until lightly browned but not cooked through, 30 seconds to 1 minute more. Transfer to a plate.

- Step 4

Add bok choy and broth to the pan. Cover and cook until the bok choy greens are bright green and almost all the liquid has been absorbed, 1 to 2 minutes. Return the beef to the pan, add the reserved sauce, and stir-fry until the beef is just cooked through and the bok choy is tender-crisp, 30 seconds to 1 minute.

Peppery Barbecue-Glazed Shrimp with Vegetables & Orzo

Ingredients

- 1 pound peeled and deveined jumbo shrimp, thawed if frozen (see Tip)

- 1 teaspoon paprika

- ½ teaspoon garlic powder

- ½ teaspoon dried oregano, crushed

- ¼ teaspoon ground pepper

- ⅛ teaspoon cayenne pepper

- 1 cup whole-grain orzo

- 3 scallions

- 2 tablespoons olive oil, divided

- 2 cups coarsely chopped zucchini

- 1 cup coarsely chopped bell pepper

- ½ cup thinly sliced celery

- 1 cup cherry tomatoes, halved

- ½ teaspoon salt

- 2 tablespoons barbecue sauce

- Lemon wedges for serving

Directions

- Step 1

Place shrimp in a medium bowl. Combine paprika, garlic powder, oregano, pepper and cayenne in a small bowl. Sprinkle the spice mixture over the shrimp; toss to coat and set aside.

- Step 2

Bring a large saucepan of water to a boil. Cook orzo according to package directions; drain. Return to the hot pot; cover and keep warm.

- Step 3

Meanwhile, slice scallions, separating white and green parts. Heat 1 tablespoon oil in a medium skillet over medium-high heat. Add the scallion whites, zucchini, bell pepper and celery; cook, stirring occasionally, until the vegetables are crisp-tender, about 5 minutes. Add tomatoes; cook until softened, 2 to 3 minutes more. Add the vegetables to the pot with the orzo. Add salt; toss to combine.

- Step 4

In same skillet, heat the remaining 1 tablespoon oil over medium heat. Add the shrimp; cook, turning once, until opaque, 4 to 6 minutes. Drizzle with barbecue sauce. Cook and stir until the shrimp are coated, about 1 minute.

- Step 5

Serve the shrimp with the vegetable mixture. Top with scallion greens and serve with lemon wedges, if desired.

Mushroom-Swiss Turkey Burgers

Ingredients

- 2 tablespoons extra-virgin olive oil

- 1 clove garlic, minced

- ¾ teaspoon ground pepper, divided

- ½ teaspoon salt, divided

- 8 portobello mushroom caps, stems and gills removed (see Tips)

- 1 pound lean ground turkey

- 2 teaspoons gluten-free Worcestershire sauce

- 1 teaspoon Dijon mustard

- 4 slices Swiss cheese

- 1 small tomato, thinly sliced

- 3 cups baby arugula

Directions

- Step 1

Preheat grill to medium-high (400-450 degrees F). Combine oil, garlic and 1/4 teaspoon each pepper and salt in a small bowl. Brush portobello caps with the oil mixture; set aside to marinate at room temperature for 10 minutes.

- Step 2

Meanwhile, combine ground turkey, Worcestershire, mustard and the remaining 1/2 teaspoon pepper and 1/4 teaspoon salt in a medium bowl. Gently mix to incorporate. (Do not overmix.) Shape into four 3/4-inch-thick patties and set aside.

- Step 3

Oil the grill rack (see Tips). Place the mushrooms, cap-side down, on the oiled grill rack. Grill, covered, until just tender, about 4 minutes per side. Transfer the mushrooms to a plate; cover to keep warm. Oil the rack again; place the turkey patties on the oiled rack. Grill, covered, until the patties are lightly charred and an instant-read thermometer inserted in the center registers 165 degrees F, 4 to 5 minutes per side. Place 1 cheese slice on each patty during the last minute of cooking. Transfer the patties to a plate and let rest for 5 minutes. (If your grill is large enough, grill the portobello caps and the patties at the same time.)

• Step 4

Place each patty on the stem side of a portobello cap; top evenly with tomato slices and arugula. Cover with the remaining portobello caps, stem-side down, and serve immediately.

Sheet-Pan Chili-Lime Salmon with Potatoes & Peppers

Ingredients

• 1 pound Yukon Gold potatoes, cut into 3/4-inch pieces

• 2 tablespoons extra-virgin olive oil, divided

• ¾ teaspoon salt, divided

• ¼ teaspoon ground pepper

- 2 teaspoons chili powder

- 1 teaspoon ground cumin

- ½ teaspoon garlic powder

- 1 lime, zested and quartered

- 2 medium bell peppers, any color, sliced

- 1 ¼ pounds center-cut salmon fillet, skinned, if desired, and cut into 4 portions

Directions

- Step 1

Preheat oven to 425 degrees F. Coat a large rimmed baking sheet with cooking spray.

- Step 2

Toss potatoes, 1 tablespoon oil, 1/4 teaspoon salt and pepper together in a medium bowl. Transfer to the prepared pan and roast for 15 minutes.

- Step 3

Meanwhile, combine chili powder, cumin, garlic powder, lime zest and the remaining 1/2 teaspoon salt in a small bowl. Place bell peppers in the medium bowl and add the remaining 1 tablespoon oil and 1/2 tablespoon of the spice mixture; toss well to coat. Coat the salmon with the remaining spice mixture.

- Step 4

After 15 minutes, remove the pan from the oven. Add the peppers and stir to combine. Roast for 5 minutes. Remove from the oven; move some of the vegetables over and add the salmon to the pan. Roast until the salmon is just cooked through, 6 to 8 minutes. Serve with lime wedges.

Baked Halibut with Brussels Sprouts & Quinoa

Ingredients

- 1 pound Brussels sprouts, trimmed and sliced

- 1 fennel bulb, trimmed and cut into strips

- 1 tablespoon plus 1 teaspoon olive oil, divided

- ½ teaspoon salt, divided

- ½ teaspoon ground pepper, divided

- 1 (1 pound) halibut fillet, cut into 4 portions

- 4 cloves garlic, minced, divided

- 3 tablespoons lemon juice

- 2 tablespoons unsalted butter, melted

- 2 cups cooked quinoa (see Associated Recipes)

- ¼ cup chopped sun-dried tomatoes

- ¼ cup chopped pitted Kalamata olives

- 2 tablespoons chopped fresh Italian parsley or fennel fronds

Directions

- Step 1

Position racks in upper and lower thirds of oven; preheat to 400 degrees F.

- Step 2

Combine Brussels sprouts, fennel, 1 Tbsp. oil, and 1/4 tsp. each salt and pepper in a large bowl; toss to coat. Spread in a single layer on a large rimmed baking sheet. Bake, stirring occasionally, until tender, 20 to 25 minutes.

- Step 3

Meanwhile, place halibut on another large rimmed baking sheet and top with half of the garlic and the remaining 1/4 tsp. each salt and pepper. Combine lemon juice and melted butter in a small bowl. Drizzle or brush half of the mixture over the fish. Bake until the fish is opaque and flakes easily with a fork, 12 to 15 minutes.

- Step 4

Meanwhile, combine quinoa, the remaining 1 tsp. oil, sun-dried tomatoes, olives, and parsley (or fennel fronds) in a medium bowl.

- Step 5

Add the remaining garlic to the lemon-butter mixture. Pour the mixture over the vegetables and bake for 1 minute more. Serve the halibut and vegetables alongside the quinoa mixture.

Vegetarian Lo Mein with Shiitakes, Carrots & Bean Sprouts

Ingredients

- 8 ounces fresh lo mein noodles or fresh or dried linguine pasta

- 2 teaspoons toasted sesame oil

- 3 tablespoons reduced-sodium soy sauce

- 2 teaspoons Sriracha

- 2 tablespoons vegetable oil, divided

- 2 tablespoons minced garlic

- 1 large carrot, halved lengthwise and cut into 1/4-inch-thick half-moon slices (about 1 cup)

- 4 ounces fresh shiitake mushrooms, stems removed, caps sliced 1/4-inch thick

- 1 cup thinly sliced celery

- 2 cups bean sprouts

- 3 tablespoons finely chopped fresh cilantro

Directions

- Step 1

Bring a large pot of water to a boil. Cook noodles according to package directions. Drain, rinse with cold water, and shake out excess water until the noodles are completely dry (pat noodles dry if needed). Transfer to a large bowl and toss with sesame oil; set aside. Combine soy sauce and Sriracha in a small bowl; set aside.

- Step 2

Heat a 14-inch flat-bottomed carbon-steel wok (or 12-inch stainless-steel skillet) over high heat until a drop of water vaporizes within 1 to 2 seconds of contact. Swirl in 1 Tbsp. vegetable oil. Add garlic; stir-fry until just fragrant, about 10 seconds. Add carrot, mushrooms, and celery; stir-fry until the celery is bright green and the vegetables have absorbed all the oil, about 1 minute.

- Step 3

Swirl in the remaining 1 Tbsp. vegetable oil. Add bean sprouts, the noodles, and the soy sauce mixture; stir-fry until the noodles are heated through and the vegetables are tender-crisp, 1 to 2 minutes. Add cilantro and toss to combine.

Charred Shrimp, Pesto & Quinoa Bowls

Ingredients

- ⅓ cup prepared pesto

- 2 tablespoons balsamic vinegar

- 1 tablespoon extra-virgin olive oil

- ½ teaspoon salt

- ¼ teaspoon ground pepper

- 1 pound peeled and deveined large shrimp (16-20 count), patted dry

- 4 cups arugula

- 2 cups cooked quinoa

- 1 cup halved cherry tomatoes

- 1 avocado, diced

Directions

- Step 1

Whisk pesto, vinegar, oil, salt and pepper in a large bowl. Remove 4 tablespoons of the mixture to a small bowl; set both bowls aside.

- Step 2

Heat a large cast-iron skillet over medium-high heat. Add shrimp and cook, stirring, until just cooked through with a slight char, 4 to 5 minutes. Remove to a plate.

- Step 3

Add arugula and quinoa to the large bowl with the vinaigrette and toss to coat. Divide the arugula mixture between 4 bowls. Top with tomatoes, avocado and shrimp. Drizzle each bowl with 1 tablespoon of the reserved pesto mixture.

Sweet & Spicy Roasted Salmon with Wild Rice Pilaf

Ingredients

- 5 skinless salmon fillets, fresh or frozen (1 1/4 lbs.)

- 2 tablespoons balsamic vinegar

- 1 tablespoon honey

- ¼ teaspoon salt

- ⅛ teaspoon ground pepper

- 1 cup chopped red and/or yellow bell pepper

- ½ to 1 small jalapeño pepper, seeded and finely chopped

- 2 scallions (green parts only), thinly sliced

- ¼ cup chopped fresh Italian parsley

- 2 2/3 cups Wild Rice Pilaf (see Associated Recipes)

Directions

- Step 1

Thaw salmon, if frozen. Preheat oven to 425 degrees F. Line a 15-by-10-inch baking pan with parchment paper. Place the salmon in the prepared pan. Whisk vinegar and honey in a small bowl; drizzle half of the mixture over the salmon. Sprinkle with salt and pepper.

- Step 2

Roast the salmon until the thickest part flakes easily, about 15 minutes. Drizzle with the remaining vinegar mixture.

- Step 3

Coat a 10-inch nonstick skillet with cooking spray; heat over medium heat. Add bell pepper and jalapeño; cook, stirring frequently, just until tender, 3 to 5 minutes. Remove from heat. Stir in scallion greens.

- Step 4

Top 4 of the salmon fillets with the pepper mixture and parsley. Serve with pilaf. (Refrigerate the remaining salmon for another use, see Note.)

Zucchini-Chickpea Veggie Burgers with Tahini-Ranch Sauce

Ingredients

- 4 tablespoons tahini, divided

- 1 tablespoon lemon juice

- 3 teaspoons white miso, divided

- 1 ¼ teaspoons onion powder, divided

- 1 ¼ teaspoons garlic powder, divided

- 1 ¼ teaspoons ground pepper, divided

- 2 tablespoons water

- 1 teaspoon chopped fresh chives plus 2 tablespoons, divided

- 1 (15 ounce) can no-salt-added chickpeas, rinsed

- 1 teaspoon ground cumin

- ¼ teaspoon salt

- ¼ cup fresh parsley leaves

- ½ cup shredded zucchini

- ⅓ cup old-fashioned rolled oats

- 1 tablespoon extra-virgin olive oil

- 4 whole-grain hamburger buns, toasted

- 1 cup packed fresh arugula

- 4 slices tomato

Directions

- Step 1

Combine 2 tablespoons tahini, lemon juice, 1 teaspoon miso, 1/2 teaspoon onion powder, 1/4 teaspoon garlic powder and 1/4 teaspoon pepper in a small bowl. Gradually whisk in water until the mixture is smooth. Stir in 1 teaspoon chives. Set aside.

- Step 2

Place chickpeas, cumin, salt and the remaining 2 tablespoons tahini, 2 teaspoons miso, 1 teaspoon garlic powder, 1 teaspoon pepper and 3/4 teaspoon onion powder in a food processor. Pulse, stopping once or twice to scrape down the sides, until a coarse mixture forms that holds together when pressed. Add parsley and the remaining 2 tablespoons chives; pulse until the herbs are finely chopped and incorporated into the mixture. Transfer to a bowl.

- Step 3

Squeeze zucchini in a clean kitchen towel to remove extra moisture. Add the zucchini and oats to the chickpea mixture; use your hands to combine, pressing to mash together. Form into 4 patties.

- Step 4

Heat oil in a large nonstick skillet over medium-high heat. Add the patties and cook until golden and beginning to crisp, 4 to 5 minutes. Carefully flip and cook until golden brown, 2 to 4 minutes more.

- Step 5

Serve the burgers on buns with the tahini-ranch sauce, arugula and tomato slices.

Lemon-Tahini Couscous with Chicken & Vegetables

Ingredients

- 1 cup whole-wheat pearl couscous (see Tip)

- ¼ cup tahini

- ¼ cup water

- 2 teaspoons lemon zest

- 2 tablespoons lemon juice

- 2 tablespoons olive oil, divided

- ½ teaspoon salt

- ¼ teaspoon ground pepper

- ¼ teaspoon crushed red pepper

- 1 clove garlic, minced

- 2 cups sliced mushrooms (half of a 10-oz. package)

- ½ medium red bell pepper, chopped

- 4 cups coleslaw mix (half of a 12- to 14-oz. package)

- 4 cups baby spinach (half of a 5-oz. bag)

- 12 ounces cooked chicken breast, chopped (about 2 1/2 cups)

- ¼ cup toasted sliced almonds

- ¼ cup crumbled reduced-fat feta cheese

- 1 tablespoon chopped fresh parsley

- 1 lemon, cut into wedges (Optional)

Directions

- Step 1

Cook couscous in a medium saucepan according to package directions. Fluff with a fork and set aside.

- Step 2

Meanwhile, whisk tahini, water, lemon juice, 1 Tbsp. oil, salt, pepper, and crushed red pepper in a small bowl until well blended; set aside.

- Step 3

Heat the remaining 1 Tbsp. oil in a large nonstick skillet over medium-high heat. Add garlic and cook until fragrant, about

30 seconds. Add mushrooms and bell pepper; cook until the mushrooms release their liquid, about 3 minutes.

- Step 4

Stir in coleslaw mix and spinach; continue cooking, stirring, until the spinach wilts, about 2 minutes. Stir in chicken, the couscous, and the tahini sauce; cook until heated through, 2 to 4 minutes.

- Step 5

Sprinkle with almonds, feta, parsley, and lemon zest. Serve with lemon wedges, if desired.

Big Beautiful Summer Salad

Ingredients

- 3 small golden beets (10 ounces total), peeled and trimmed

- 2 small ripe avocados (6 ounces each)

- 1 cup chopped fresh herbs (such as tarragon, dill, parsley, chives and/or cilantro)

- ½ cup plus 2 tablespoons low-fat buttermilk

- 2 tablespoons water

- 1 small garlic clove

- 2 tablespoons plus 4 teaspoons fresh lemon juice, divided

- ¾ teaspoon salt, divided

- 8 cups chopped romaine lettuce

- 1 (15.5 ounce) can no-salt-added chickpeas, drained and rinsed

- 1 cup lightly packed microgreens (such as pea shoots)

- 1 cup fresh corn kernels (from 2 ears)

- 1 cup frozen edamame, thawed

- 1 small watermelon radish, halved and thinly sliced on a mandoline (about 1/4 cup)

- 2 tablespoons extra-virgin olive oil

Directions

- Step 1

Wrap beets together in 1 sheet of microwavable parchment paper. Microwave on High until tender, 10 to 12 minutes. Let cool for 5 minutes. Cut each beet into 8 wedges.

- Step 2

Meanwhile, cut 1 avocado into 12 wedges. Chop the remaining avocado.

- Step 3

Combine herbs, buttermilk, water, garlic, 2 tablespoons plus 2 teaspoons lemon juice and 1/4 teaspoon salt in a blender. Puree until smooth, about 10 seconds, stopping to scrape down sides as needed. Add the chopped avocado; process on medium speed until blended and smooth, about 30 seconds, stopping to scrape down sides as needed.

- Step 4

Arrange romaine on a large platter. Top with chickpeas, microgreens, corn, edamame, radish slices, beet wedges and avocado wedges. Drizzle with oil and the remaining 2 teaspoons lemon juice; sprinkle with the remaining 1/2 teaspoon salt. Spoon the buttermilk dressing over the salad.

Tofu Tacos

Ingredients

- 1 tablespoon chili powder

- 1 teaspoon ground cumin

- ½ teaspoon dried oregano

- ½ teaspoon salt

- ¼ teaspoon ground pepper

- ⅛ teaspoon ground cinnamon

- 1 (14 to 16 ounce) block extra-firm tofu, patted dry and cut into 1/2-inch pieces

- 3 tablespoons extra-virgin olive oil, divided

- ½ cup chopped onion

* 2 large cloves garlic, minced

* 1 (15 ounce) can black beans, rinsed

* 2 teaspoons cider vinegar

* ½ cup chopped cilantro

* 8 corn tortillas, warmed

* ¼ cup Shredded cabbage, pico de gallo and/or guacamole

Directions

* Step 1

Combine chili powder, cumin, oregano, salt, pepper and cinnamon in a medium bowl. Add tofu and toss to coat. Set aside.

* Step 2

Heat 2 tablespoons oil in a large nonstick skillet over medium heat. Add onion; cook, stirring, until starting to soften, about 3 minutes. Add garlic; cook, stirring, for 1 minute. Increase heat to medium-high and add tofu; cook, stirring occasionally, until starting to brown, about 10 minutes. Add beans; cook, stirring, until heated through, 2 to 3 minutes. Remove from heat; stir in vinegar and cilantro.

- Step 3

To serve, fill each tortilla with about 1/3 cup tofu filling. Top with cabbage, pico de gallo and/or guacamole, if desired.

Chile-Lime Tilapia with Corn Sauté

Ingredients

- 4 4-5 ounce fresh or frozen skinless white firm-fleshed fish fillets, such as tilapia, catfish, sole, flounder, or cod

- 1 tablespoon lime juice

- 1 ½ teaspoon ground ancho chile pepper or chili powder

- ¼ teaspoon salt

- 1 tablespoon canola oil

- 2 0.667 cup frozen whole kernel roasted or regular corn, thawed

- ¼ cup finely chopped red onion

- 2 teaspoon finely chopped seeded fresh jalapeño chile pepper*

- 2 cloves garlic, minced

- 1 tablespoon snipped fresh cilantro

- Lime wedges and/or additional jalapeño slices (optional)

Directions

1. Thaw fish, if frozen. Rinse fish; pat dry. Measure thickness of fish. In a bowl stir together lime juice, ancho chile pepper,

and salt. Brush lime mixture evenly over both sides of fish fillets.

2. In an extra-large nonstick skillet heat 2 tsp. of the oil over medium-high heat. Add fish; cook 4 to 6 minutes per 1/2-inch thickness or until fish flakes easily, turning once. Remove fish from skillet. Cover and keep warm.

3. In the same skillet heat the remaining 1 tsp. oil. Add the next four ingredients (through garlic); cook about 2 minutes or until vegetables are heated and are just starting to soften, stirring occasionally. Remove from heat.

4. Divide corn mixture among plates. Top with fish and sprinkle with cilantro. If desired, serve with lime wedges and/or additional jalapeño slices.

Seared Salmon with Pistachio Gremolata

Ingredients

- ⅓ cup roasted salted pistachio nuts, finely chopped

- ⅓ cup chopped fresh parsley

- 2 tablespoon chopped fresh mint

- 1 tablespoon orange zest

- 1 tablespoon olive oil

- 2 cloves garlic, minced

- ⅛ teaspoon salt

- 1 tablespoon olive oil

- 1 pound salmon fillet, skinned and cut into 4 pieces

- ¼ teaspoon salt

- ¼ teaspoon black pepper

Directions

1. For pistachio gremolata, in a small bowl combine the first seven ingredients (through 1/8 teaspoon salt).

2. In a very large skillet heat 1 Tbsp. olive oil over medium-high heat. Season salmon with 1/4 tsp. each salt and pepper. Carefully place salmon in skillet. Cook 3 minutes. Turn and cook 3 minutes more or just until salmon flakes. Top with pistachio gremolata.

Balsamic Chicken and Vegetables

Ingredients

- ¼ cup bottled Italian salad dressing

- 2 tablespoon balsamic vinegar

- 1 tablespoon honey

- ⅛ - ¼ teaspoon crushed red pepper

- 2 tablespoon olive oil

- 1 pound chicken breast tenderloins

- 10 ounce fresh asparagus, trimmed and cut into 2-inch pieces, or one 10-ounce package frozen cut asparagus, thawed and well drained

- 1 cup purchased shredded carrot

- 1 small tomato, seeded and chopped

Directions

1. In a small bowl, stir together salad dressing, balsamic vinegar, honey, and crushed red pepper. Set aside.

2. In a large skillet, heat oil over medium-high heat. Add chicken; cook for 5 to 6 minutes or until chicken is tender and no longer pink, turning once. Add half of the dressing mixture to skillet; turn chicken to coat. Transfer chicken to a serving platter; cover and keep warm.

3. Add asparagus and carrot to skillet. Cook and stir for 3 to 4 minutes or until asparagus is crisp-tender; transfer to serving platter.

4. Stir remaining dressing mixture; add to skillet. Cook and stir for 1 minute, scraping up browned bits from bottom of skillet. Drizzle the dressing mixture over chicken and vegetables. Sprinkle with tomato. Makes 4 servings.

Skillet Lasagna

Ingredients

• Nonstick cooking spray

• 8 ounce ground turkey or extra-lean ground beef (93% lean)*

• ¾ cup chopped green, red, or yellow sweet pepper

- ½ cup chopped onion

- 2 cloves garlic, minced

- 1 23.5 ounce jar light traditional-flavored pasta sauce, such as Prego Heart Smart

- 1 cup water

- 2 cup packaged sliced fresh mushrooms

- 3 cup dried wide egg noodles

- ½ cup light ricotta cheese

- 2 tablespoon grated Parmesan or Romano cheese

- ½ teaspoon dried Italian seasoning, crushed

- ½ cup shredded part-skim mozzarella cheese (2 oz.)

Directions

1. Coat an extra-large nonstick skillet with cooking spray; heat skillet over medium heat. Cook beef, sweet pepper, onion, and garlic until meat is browned; stirring to break up meat as it cooks. Drain off any fat. Stir in pasta sauce and water. Bring to boiling. Add mushrooms and uncooked noodles; stir to separate noodles. Return to boiling; reduce heat. Cover and gently boil about 10 minutes or until pasta is tender, stirring occasionally.

2. Meanwhile, in a bowl stir together ricotta, Parmesan, and Italian seasoning. Drop cheese mixture by spoonfuls into 10 small mounds (about 1 tablespoon each) on top pasta mixture in skillet. Sprinkle each mound with mozzarella. Reduce heat to low. Cook, covered, 4 to 5 minutes or until cheese mixture is

heated and mozzarella is melted. Serve immediately.

Veggie Tostadas with Cauliflower Mash

Ingredients

- 2 cup cauliflower florets

- ¼ cup Mexican Crema or sour cream

- 2 tablespoon coconut oil or olive oil

- 1 teaspoon salt

- 1 teaspoon chopped canned chipotle pepper in adobo sauce

- 1 cup bite-size pieces fresh asparagus

- 1 cup frozen whole kernel corn

- 1 cup quartered grape tomatoes

- 8 tostada shells

- ¼ cup crumbled queso blanco or feta cheese (1 oz.)

Directions

1. In a covered large saucepan steam cauliflower, covered, in a steamer basket over a small amount of boiling water 4 minutes or until fork-tender. Transfer cauliflower to a food processor. Add Mexican Crema, 1 Tbsp. of the oil, 1/2 tsp. of the salt, and the chipotle pepper. Cover and process until smooth.

2. In covered saucepan steam asparagus and corn in basket over boiling water 5 to 7 minutes or until tender; drain and return to saucepan. Add tomatoes and remaining 1 Tbsp. oil and 1/2 tsp. salt; toss to coat.

3. Spread tostada shells with cauliflower mixture and top with asparagus mixture. Sprinkle with queso blanco.

Spicy Shrimp Pasta

Ingredients

• 12 ounce fresh or frozen large shrimp in shells

• 8 ounce dried linguine or fettuccine

• 2 tablespoon olive oil or vegetable oil

• 1 - 2 fresh jalapeño chile peppers, finely chopped

• 2 cloves garlic, minced

• ½ teaspoon salt

• ¼ teaspoon ground black pepper

• 2 cup cherry tomatoes, halved

• Finely shredded Parmesan cheese (optional)

Directions

1. Thaw shrimp, if frozen. Peel and devein shrimp. Rinse shrimp; pat dry

with paper towels. In a large saucepan cook linguine according to package directions; drain. Return linguine to hot saucepan; cover and keep warm.

2. Meanwhile, in a large skillet heat oil over medium-high heat. Add chile peppers, garlic, salt, and black pepper; cook and stir for 1 minute. Add shrimp; cook and stir about 3 minutes or until shrimp are opaque. Stir in tomatoes; heat through.

3. Add shrimp mixture to cooked linguine; gently toss to combine. If desired, serve with cheese.

Cilantro-Ginger Chicken with Peanuts

Ingredients

- 2 teaspoon peanut oil

- 1 pound skinless, boneless chicken breast halves, cut into 1-inch pieces

- ¼ cup honey-roasted peanuts

- 2 - 3 teaspoon minced fresh ginger

- 4 cloves garlic, minced

- ¼ cup sliced green onion

- 1 tablespoon soy sauce

- 2 teaspoon rice vinegar

- 1 teaspoon toasted sesame oil

- 1 cup fresh cilantro leaves

- 4 cup finely shredded napa cabbage or 2 cups hot cooked brown rice

- Lime wedges (optional)

Directions

1. In a large heavy skillet heat peanut oil over medium-high heat. Add chicken; cook and stir 2 minutes. Add peanuts,

ginger, and garlic; cook and stir 3 minutes or until chicken is no longer pink.

2. Add green onions, soy sauce, vinegar, and sesame oil to skillet. Cook and stir 2 minutes more. Remove from heat. Stir in cilantro.

3. Serve chicken mixture over cabbage. If desired, top with additional cilantro and serve with lime wedges.

Quick Eggplant Parmigiana

Ingredients

- 1 small eggplant (12 oz.)

- 1 egg, lightly beaten

- 1 tablespoon water

- ¼ cup all-purpose flour

- 2 tablespoon vegetable oil

- ⅓ cup grated Parmesan cheese

- 1 cup meatless spaghetti sauce

- ¾ cup shredded mozzarella cheese (3 oz.)

- Fresh basil (optional)

Directions

1. Peel eggplant; cut crosswise into 1/2-inch slices. Combine egg and the water. Dip eggplant slices into egg mixture, then into flour, turning to coat.

2. In a 10-inch skillet heat oil over medium-high. Add eggplant, half at a time, and cook 4 to 6 minutes or until golden, turning once. (If needed, add additional oil and reduce heat to medium if eggplant browns too quickly.) Drain on paper towels.

3. Wipe skillet with paper towels. Arrange eggplant slices in skillet;

sprinkle with Parmesan cheese. Top with spaghetti sauce and mozzarella cheese. Cook, covered, over medium-low heat 5 to 7 minutes or until heated through. If desired, top with additional Parmesan cheese and basil.

Salmon with Lemon and Herbs

Ingredients

- ⅔ cup mayonnaise

- 1 ½ teaspoon lemon zest

- 1 tablespoon lemon juice

- 1 clove garlic, minced

- 2 tablespoon minced fresh chives

- 2 teaspoon finely chopped fresh tarragon

- 2 teaspoon finely chopped fresh parsley

- ¼ teaspoon sugar

- Kosher salt

- Black pepper

- 2 - 2 ½ pound center cut salmon fillet, skin on

- Thin lemon slices and/or parsley leaves (optional)

Directions

1. Preheat oven to 450°F. For sauce, a bowl combine the first eight ingredients (through sugar). Season mixture to taste with salt and pepper.

2. Place salmon on a foil-lined baking sheet. Measure thickness of fish. Season with salt and pepper. Spread 1/4 cup sauce over top of salmon. Roast 4 to 6 minutes per 1/2-inch thickness of fish or just until fish flakes when tested with a fork. Let rest 5 minutes.

3. Add water, 1 tsp. at a time, to remaining sauce to thin to desired consistency. Serve salmon with sauce. If desired, top with several thin lemon slices and/or sprinkle with parsley.

SUMMARY

As new evidence emerges, the link between diet and heart disease grows stronger.

What you eat can influence almost every aspect of heart health, from blood pressure and inflammation to cholesterol levels and triglycerides.

Including these heart-healthy foods as part of a nutritious, well-balanced diet can help keep your heart in good shape and minimize your risk of heart disease.

Studies show that your diet can either increase or decrease your risk of developing heart disease.

While diets high in ultra-processed foods and added sugar have been associated with increased risk, dietary patterns high in fiber-rich plant foods like fruits and vegetables, fish, and healthy fats like olive oil can support heart health.

Whether you're living with heart disease or simply trying to reduce your risk of developing cardiovascular disease in the future, making a few simple dietary changes can have a profound effect on your heart health.